MW01290636

Vegan Cookbook for Beginners
Transform Your Life!

Fat-Free Quick & Easy Vegan Recipes
Delicious Recipes Purely Starch-Plant Based for a
Dairy-Free, Low-Cholesterol, Low-Fat Diet

Series: Low-Fat Vegan Cooking Recipe Book (3)

By Anna I. Jäger
Co-Author: Holly Tomlinson

ISBN-13: 978-1523606726
ISBN-10: 152360672X

Content

Introduction

Eating a whole-foods diet without animal foods and without added oils, less salt and sugar, and very few processed foods dramatically improves the health!
The recipes in this book are based on a purely starch-plant based diet (diet based on whole starches, vegetables, and fruits) without added oils. Cheers to you for bidding goodbye to animal products, to processed foods and to oil! Consume only fats that are still in their natural packaging—such as in whole foods.

The recommended low-fat vegan diet is based on scientific research and recommendations by experts such as Dr. Neal Barnard, T. Collin Campbell, Michael McGregor, and Dr. John McDougall.

If you are ready to transform your life and enjoy some delicious vegan recipes, keep reading!

35 Recipes: Menu Ideas for One Week
Mix and Match as You Like!

So, you've switched over to a vegan, no-fat diet. Now what? Many times when people make a decision to change their eating habits, the change is short-lived because they get bored or run out of options. This book has been designed to provide you a seven-day meal plan. The recipes within can be mixed and matched to create delicious, healthy, fat-free vegan meals.

The benefits of a vegan, fat-free, plant-based, whole foods diet are vast. Not only will this diet help those who are looking to lose weight, but it is extremely helpful for those suffering from diabetes.

There are recipes for Breakfast, Snacks, Lunch, Dinner and even healthier options for Desserts. **All the recipes are quick and easy.** Even better yet, **each category features two recipes that can be made in fifteen minutes or less or only require five ingredients or less.**

Breakfast

1| *Blueberry Pancakes*

Servings: 6-8 Pancakes

Prep Time: 4 minutes
Cook Time: 10 minutes

These pancakes are incredibly easy to make (less than fifteen minutes) and are just as incredibly delicious. You can eat them as-is or add some applesauce as a topping. Whip up a batch for some friends and see if they believe that they are vegan.

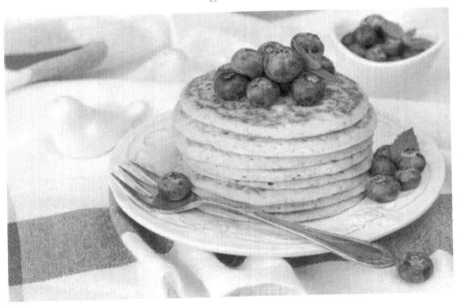

Ingredients:

- 1 cup whole wheat pastry flower
- 1 tablespoon sugar (you can use your preferred type of sugar or sweetener)
- 2 tablespoons baking powder
- 1 dash of sea salt
- 1 cup rice milk

- Blueberries to taste

Instructions:

1. Set out all your ingredients. Place a pan on the stove over medium heat.
2. Combine all your dry ingredients. Add the rice milk to the mixture and beat until smooth.
3. Spoon the mixture onto the pan. When bubbles begin to appear on the surface, flip the pancake over. Cook until it is brown on both sides.
4. Repeat until all the mixture has been used.

Tip: These can be made in large batches and frozen. Just pop them in the microwave when you are ready to eat.

Nutritional Information: 400 calories per serving, 65g carbs, 0g fat, 10g protein, 2.4g fiber

2| *French Toast*

Servings: 6

Prep Time: 5 Minutes
Cook Time: 10 Minutes

Who can resist the aroma of French toast? My recipe will allow you to indulge in this classic breakfast dish and not have all the guilt afterwards or spend all morning making them. Fifteen minutes tops! Oh, and as an added bonus...your kids will be looking for seconds.

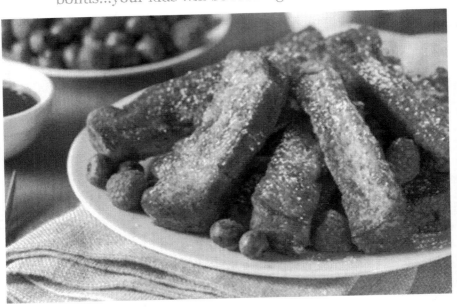

Ingredients:

- 1 cup original almond smooth milk
- ½ cup orange juice
- 2 tablespoons flour
- 1 tablespoon nutritional yeast
- ½ teaspoon cinnamon
- ¼ teaspoon nutmeg

- 6 slices of whole wheat bread

Instructions:

1. Preheat a non-stick skillet over high heat.
2. Add all ingredients to a bowl and mix together.
3. Dip a slice of bread into the mixture and place onto the skillet. Cook for about three minutes on each side.
4. Repeat until you have used all of the mixture and/or bread.
5. Serve and enjoy.

Tip: If you do not use up all of the mixture, you can store it in the fridge for use at a later time. The mixture will keep for up to five days. Also, if you have extra toasts left over, you can always save them to have later on in the day as a snack. All you have to do is toast them. They are great either plain or with a topping such as bananas or peanut butter.

Nutritional Information: 95 calories per serving, 16.6g carbs, 1.1g fat, 4.8g protein, 2.5g fiber

3| *Cinnamon Berry Oatmeal*

Servings: 2

Prep Time: 5 Minutes
Cook Time: 20 Minutes

There is nothing more comforting than a nice warm bowl of oatmeal in the morning. This oatmeal is especially wonderful because it is naturally sweet and so healthy.

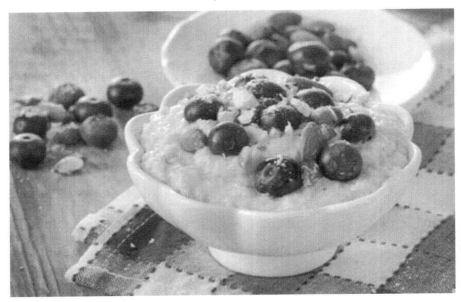

Ingredients:

- 1 cup water
- 1 teaspoon vanilla extract
- 1/4 teaspoon cinnamon
- 1/2 cup old fashioned rolled oats
- 1/2 cup blueberries (fresh or frozen)
- 2 apples, peeled, cored and diced
- 2 teaspoon chopped walnuts or almonds
- 1 tablespoon ground flax seed

Instructions:

1. In a medium saucepan add the water, vanilla and cinnamon and bring to a boil over medium heat.
2. Add the oats and reduce heat to a simmer. Cook for about five minutes.
3. Once the oats have softened, stir in the berries. Continue cooking until all of it is heated through.
4. Remove the saucepan from heat. Cover and let stand 15 minutes or until it reaches the desired thickness. Once the oatmeal has thickened and you are ready to eat, add the apples, nuts and flax.

Nutritional Information: 240.7 calories per serving, 40.8g carbs, 6g fat, 17.7g protein, 6.9g fiber

4| *Spicy Southern Grits*

Servings: 2

Prep Time: 5 Minutes
Cook Time: 15 Minutes

I have to be totally honest and say that the first time I tried grits, many years ago, I hated them. They were bland and the consistency reminded me of what movies depict as "prison food". It wasn't until recently that I tasted this version of grits that I learned what they are really supposed to look and taste like. I guarantee if you've had a not-so-good grit experience in the past, this will totally change your mind.

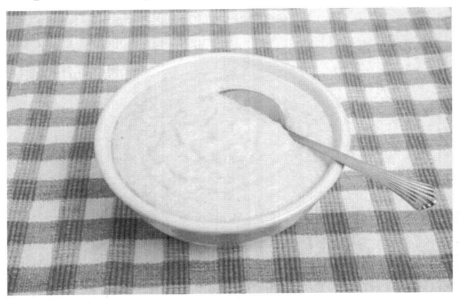

Ingredients:

- 1 small yellow onion, diced
- 1 tablespoon garlic, minced
- ¼ cup green chilies, diced

- 1 chipotle pepper, chopped
- 2 cups veggie stock
- ½ cup grits, yellow
- 3 tablespoons nutritional yeast
- ½ lime, juiced

Instructions:

1. Sautee the onions, garlic, green chilies and chipotle pepper with 2 tablespoons veggie stock for 5 to 7 minutes.
2. Add the rest of the stock and bring to a boil.
3. Using a whisk, add the grits. Turn the heat to low and cook for five minutes.
4. Stir in the nutritional yeast and the limejuice.
5. Once the grits are cooked you can add seasoning to your liking. Serve and enjoy.

Nutritional Information: 137 calories per serving, 24.8g carbs, 3g fat, 9.1g protein, 7.3g fiber

5| *Blueberry Muffins*

Servings: 1 dozen

Prep Time: 30 Minutes
Cook Time: 30 Minutes

Let's face it. We don't always have the time or desire to sit down and eat breakfast, even if it is the most important meal of the day. Cook up a batch of these muffins ahead of time and have a delicious, quick option you can have on those on-the-go days.

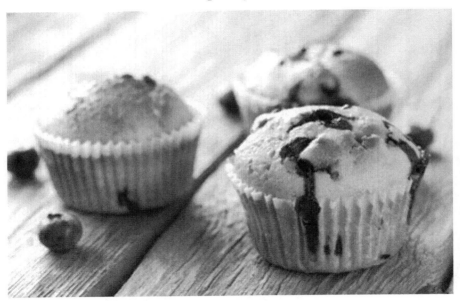

Ingredients:

- 12 dates, pitted and chopped
- 1 cup almond milk
- 1½ cups old-fashioned rolled oats
- ¾ cup dry millet
- 2 teaspoons baking powder
- ½ teaspoon ground cardamom

- ½ cup applesauce
- 1 teaspoon lemon zest, packed
- 1 cup blueberries

Instructions:

1. Preheat your oven to 350. Mix the chopped dates and the almond milk in a small bowl and set aside for about 15 to 20 minutes so that the dates can soften.
2. Using your blender, grind the oats and millet into a flour consistency. Mix the flour, baking powder and cardamom in a separate bowl and stir all the ingredients together.
3. Pour the dates and almond milk mixture into the blender and blend until it is smooth. Add the date mixture to the bowl of dry ingredients along with the applesauce and lemon zest, and mix well until all the dry ingredients have disappeared.
4. Gently fold in the blueberries. Once everything is mixed together, spoon the batter into muffin pan, filling each muffin cup about halfway full.
5. Bake the muffins for 25 to 30 minutes. You will know the muffins are ready when the tops begin to brown and cracks show up on the muffin top. You could also use the "toothpick test" to see if they are ready. Let the muffins cool for at least 15-20 minutes before removing.

Nutritional Information: 129 calories per serving, 19.8g carbs, 5g fat, 2.2g protein, 2.6g fiber

6| *Breakfast Cookies*

Servings: 12

Prep Time: 10 Minutes
Cook Time: 25 Minutes

So, you've been working hard all week to eat healthy. You deserve a treat, don't you? These breakfast cookies are exactly what you need. They are full of good stuff, so there will be no room for guilt after eating these.

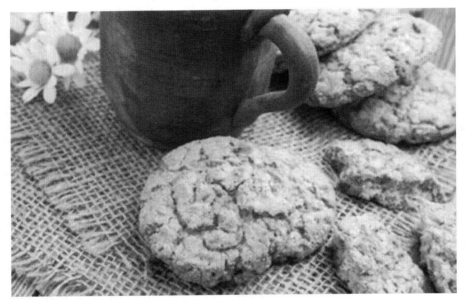

Ingredients:

- ¼ cup unsweetened applesauce
- 2 tablespoons chia seeds
- ½ cup date paste
- 1 teaspoon vanilla extract
- 2 ripe bananas, mashed
- 2 tablespoons fine chopped walnuts
- 1 cup rolled oats

- ½ cup unbleached flour
- ½ teaspoon baking soda

Instructions:

1. Preheat oven to 350 degrees.
2. Combine the applesauce, chia seeds, date paste and vanilla and bananas into a bowl and mix until smooth. Set the bowl aside so that the chia seeds can start to gel.
3. In a separate bowl, combine the walnuts and the dry ingredients. Combine the wet ingredients into this mix. Mix well with a wooden spoon.
4. Scoop the cookies onto the baking sheet. With a spatula or a knife, flatten the cookies to your desired thickness. Thicker cookies will be chewier.
5. Place in oven and bake for 23-25 minutes. Once they are ready, remove and let cool before serving.

Tip: These can be stored in an airtight container or Ziploc and frozen.

Nutritional Information: 92 calories per serving, 18.7g carbs, 1g fat, 2.1g protein, 1.7g fiber

7| *Breakfast Tortillas*

Servings: 6-8

Prep Time: 10 Minutes
Cook Time: 10 Minutes

Here's a little fancier dish that you can serve occasionally at home, or make for guests. It is very filling and something different to change things up a bit.

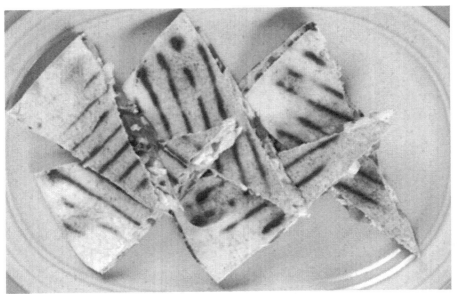

Ingredients:

- 2 cups packed spinach
- 2 cups cooked brown rice
- 1 cup frozen corn kernels
- ½ cup salsa
- 6 to 8 whole wheat or corn tortillas

Instructions:

1. Place the spinach in a saucepan. Make sure that the

leaves are wet. Cook for about two minutes, or until it is just wilted. Remove from the saucepan and drain well.
2. Place the brown rice, corn, and salsa in the saucepan. Cook until heated through and then stir in the spinach.
3. Once everything is cooked spoon some of the mixture onto each tortilla and roll.

Nutritional Information: 234 calories per serving, 49.5g carbs, 2g fat, 5.6g protein, 3.7g fiber

Snacks

Recipes Included in this Chapter:

1| *Watermelon Salad*

Servings: 4-6

Prep Time: 10 Minutes
Cook Time: 0 Minutes

This refreshing, easy to make salad can be either prepared on the spot or ahead of time. It's a great snack to have on hand whenever your sweet tooth strikes.

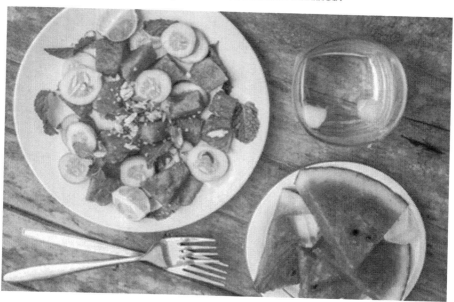

Ingredients:

- Half of a Watermelon
- 1 Cucumber
- Chopped mint
- Lime Juice

Instructions:

1. Cube and seed the watermelon and cut up the cucumber. The amount of watermelon and cucumber used is entirely up to you.
2. Add fresh mint and lime to taste.

Tip: *If you have too much of this salad left over, do not fret. Throw it into the blender with some ice and turn it into a slushy!*

Nutritional Information: 11 calories per serving, 2.6g carbs, 0g fat, 0g protein, 0g fiber

2| *Peanut Butter and Jelly Smoothie*

Servings: 1

Prep Time: 5 Minutes
Cook Time: 5 Minutes

This super easy and quick recipe is a great twist on an old favorite. Make this for yourself, for friends or for your whole family.

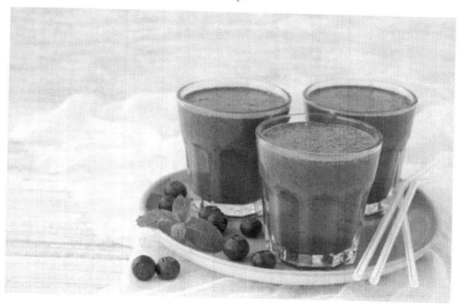

Ingredients:

- 1 Banana
- 1 cup Raspberries
- 2 Tablespoons Organic Peanut Butter (contains less fat than regular peanut butter)
- 1 ½ cups rice milk of your choosing
- Ice (if using fresh fruits)

Instructions:

1. Add all of your ingredients to the blender and blend!
2. Serve and enjoy.

Nutritional Information: 349 calories per serving, 78.9g carbs, 4.2g fat, 3.4g protein, 11g fiber

3| *Banana Blueberry Bars*

Servings: 12 bars

Prep Time: 15 Minutes
Cook Time: 35 Minutes

These tasty bars make for a wonderful snack. They are full of
healthy starches that will provide energy to last you through
until your next meal.

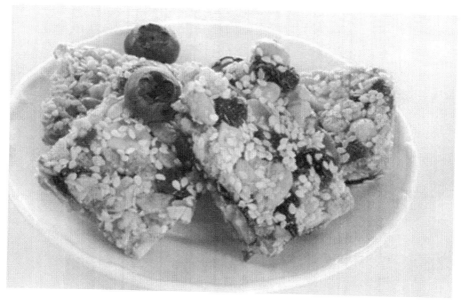

Ingredients:

- 1 cup dates, pitted and halved
- 1½ cups apple juice
- 1 cup oat flour
- 2 cups rolled oats
- ¾ teaspoon cinnamon
- ¼ teaspoon nutmeg
- 3 bananas
- 1 teaspoon pure vanilla extract

- ½ cup blueberries
- ½ cup walnuts

Instructions:

1. Preheat oven to 350°F.
2. Cover a baking pan with parchment paper.
3. Add dates and apple juice into a small bowl and allow the dates to soak for about 10-15 minutes.
4. In a separate bowl, combine flour, oats, cinnamon, and nutmeg. Mix together and set aside.
5. Place the bananas and vanilla extract into a blender. Remove dates from the apple juice and add the strained juice to the blender and blend until creamy. Now add the dates to the blender and pulse a few times until the dates are in small pieces.
6. Pour the banana mixture into bowl with the dry ingredients. Mix all of the ingredients well. Stir in the blueberries and walnuts.
7. Pour the batter into baking pan. Bake at 350°F for 30 minutes. Let cool at room temperature for 5 to 10 minutes before cutting and serving.

Nutritional Information: 202 calories per serving, 37.5g carbs, 4g fat, 4.8g protein, 4.7g fiber

4| *Vanilla Chia Pudding*

Servings: 2

Prep Time: 5 Minutes
Cook Time: 5 Minutes

This recipe will take you a total of ten minutes to prepare ahead of time. Have in your fridge to enjoy a smooth, delicious pudding when a snack attack strikes.

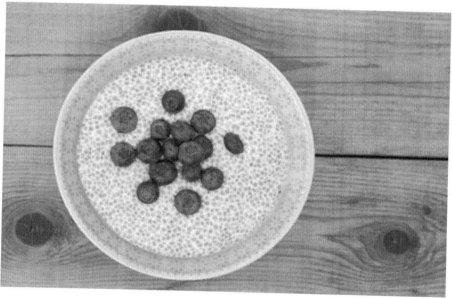

Ingredients:

- 1 cup Rice Milk
- 4 tablespoons chia seeds
- ½ teaspoon vanilla extract

Instructions:

1. Place all of your ingredients into a jar or container that can be shaken.
2. Shake well then place in the refrigerator for at least an hour or overnight.
3. Enjoy.

Nutritional Information: 63 calories per serving, 12.6g carbs, 1g fat, 0g protein, 0g fiber

5| *Apple Cookies (A healthier cookie option)*

Servings: 2

Prep Time: 5 Minutes
Cook Time: 0 Minutes

Next time that you are craving a snack, make this easy and delicious recipe. Once again, this one is great for the kids, and they won't even realize they are eating a healthier option.

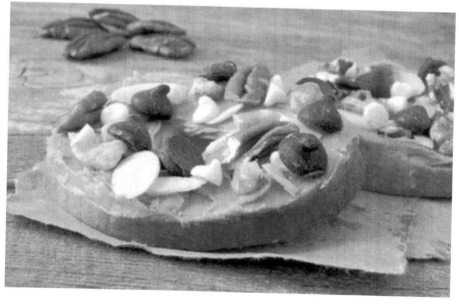

Ingredients:

- 1 apple, sliced and cored
- 2 tablespoons organic peanut butter
- Mini dairy-free chocolate chips

Instructions:

Spread peanut butter on top of the apple slices. Next

sprinkle each slice with chocolate chips. Serve and enjoy!

Tip: You can substitute the chocolate chips with shredded coconut, raisins, almonds or any other of your favorite toppings.

Nutritional Information: 47 calories per serving, 12.6g carbs, 0.2g fat, 0.2g protein, 2.2g fiber

6| *Strawberry Banana Popsicles*

Servings: 6

Prep Time: 10 Minutes

Yummy, clean-eating popsicles made with only 3 ingredients? Where can I sign up? Trust me, you will have a hard time eating just one!

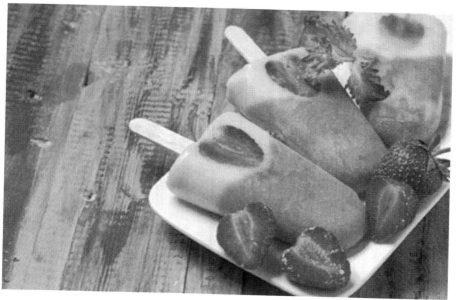

Ingredients:

- 1 large ripe banana
- 12 large strawberries, sliced in half
- ½ cup fruit juice of your choice

Note: *You will need a popsicle mold and popsicle sticks for this recipe.*

Instructions:

1. Add all of the ingredients into a blender and blend on high speed until smooth.
2. Pour the mixture into a popsicle mold. Add your popsicle sticks. (If your mold does not have slots for these you will have to freeze mixture for a couple of hours then insert the sticks and continue freezing.)
3. Let popsicles freeze overnight. Once you are ready to serve you can run the molds under warm water help remove the popsicles. Enjoy!

Tip: *Taste your mixture before freezing so that you can adjust the flavor if necessary.*

Nutritional Information: 32 calories per serving, 7.9g carbs, 0.2g fat, 0.5g protein, 1.3g fiber

7| *Baked Sweet Potato Chips*

Servings: 1-2

Prep Time: 15 Minutes
Cook Time: 12 Minutes

The perfect snack! These oil-free and easy to prepare chips
will be just what you need to satisfy your craving for salty
and crunchy.

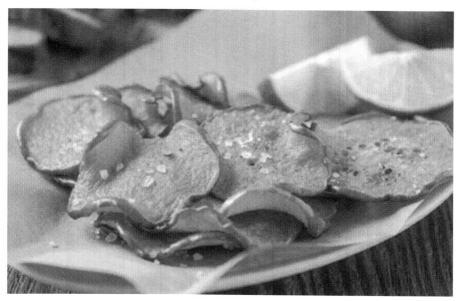

Ingredients:

- Large sweet potato
- Fine sea salt, to taste
- Seasonings of choice

Instructions:

1. Preheat oven to 400F.

2. Slice the potato into really thin slices, with or without the skin. (The use of a mandolin will be your best option, but it is not the only option.)
3. Prepare a baking sheet lined with parchment paper and arrange the slices in a single layer.
4. Sprinkle with sea salt and any other seasoning you have chosen.
5. Bake in the oven for 10 minutes. Flip each slice and continue to bake for another 2-3 minutes. Make sure to keep an eye on them because they will burn easily.

Nutritional Information: 163 calories per serving, 37.3g carbs, 0.3g fat, 3.6g protein, 6g fiber

Lunch

1| *Kale, Lemon & Cilantro Sandwich*

Servings: 2-4

Prep Time: 10 Minutes
Cook Time: 5 Minutes

This super easy and quick sandwich will have you licking your fingers. Perfect for a quick lunch that will be very filling and satisfying.

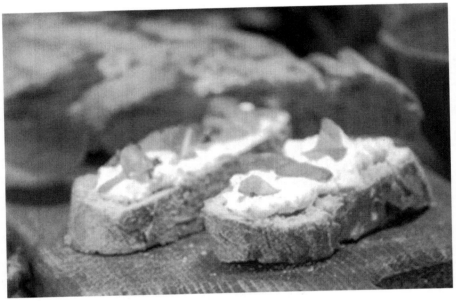

Ingredients:

- 1 bunch kale
- 4 slices whole grain bread
- Hummus
- 4 green onions
- ½ bunch cilantro
- 1 lemon sliced thinly into rounds
- Zest of 1 lemon

Instructions:

1. Tear kale leaves away from thick stem and chop into bite-size pieces. Place the kale in a pot with about 4 inches of water.
2. Bring to a boil, cover and cook until kale is tender. Check frequently.
3. Spread some hummus onto the bread and then add the green onions, cilantro and lemon rounds on top.
4. Once kale is cooked and drained well, sprinkle with the lemon zest. If you really like lemon, you can squeeze the juice of the remaining lemons on also.
5. Place a large handful of the seasoned kale onto the bread and then top with the other slice.

Nutritional Information: 78 calories per serving, 15.3g carbs, 1g fat, 3.8g protein, 2.6g fiber

2| *Pesto Pasta*

Servings: 4

Prep Time: 5 Minutes
Cook Time: 10 Minutes

I know what you're thinking – *Don't you need oil and cheese for pesto?* The answer is no! Not for this delicious recipe. Enjoy this light and fresh pasta with some vegetables.

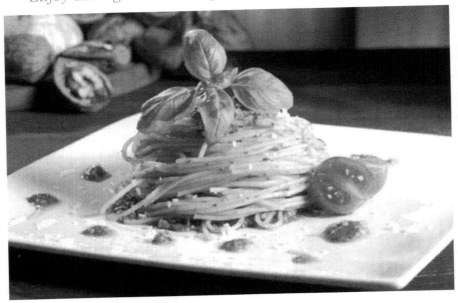

Ingredients:

- ½ cup water
- ½ cup walnuts
- ½ teaspoon minced fresh garlic (1-2 cloves)
- 1 large bunch fresh basil
- 1 package cooked whole-grain pasta of your choice

Instructions:

1. In a food processor, blend all ingredients until smooth. You can use water to thin out as needed.
2. Cook the pasta according to package directions. Once the pasta is cooked, drain.
3. Return the just-cooked pasta to its cooking pot with the heat on medium-low, and add the pesto.
4. Stir until the pasta is completely coated and the pesto is warmed through. Serve while the pesto is still warm.

Nutritional Information: 97 calories per serving, 1.7g carbs, 9g fat, 3.8g protein, 1.1g fiber

3| *Black Bean Tacos*

Servings: 8

Prep Time: 5 Minutes
Cook Time: 10 Minutes

Who doesn't love a good taco? This recipe will allow you to indulge in some delicious tacos with an amazing cilantro-lime sauce.

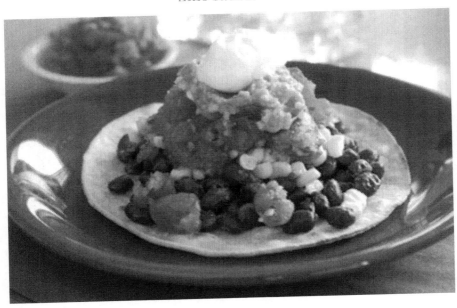

Ingredients:

- 2 cans of black beans
- 1 cup salsa
- 1 teaspoon cumin
- Corn tortillas
- Toppings of your choice
- ½ avocado
- ¾ cup cilantro (leaves only)
- 1 lime, juiced

- 1 garlic clove
- Pinch of salt

Instructions:

1. Begin by preparing the sauce. Add avocado, cilantro, limejuice, garlic and salt to a food processor. Once everything is blended, set aside.
2. Add black beans to a pan over medium heat. Add salsa and cumin. Cook for about five minutes until the beans are heated through.
3. While the beans are heating, warm up your tortillas and prepare your toppings.
4. Assemble your tacos and enjoy!

Nutritional Information: 405 calories per serving, 71g carbs, 4g fat, 24g protein, 17.8g fiber

4| *Black Beans and Rice*

Servings: 5

Prep Time: 15 Minutes
Cook Time: 10 Minutes

This dish is as basic as they come, but the flavor will tell a whole different story. Prepare this for your family or impress some friends.

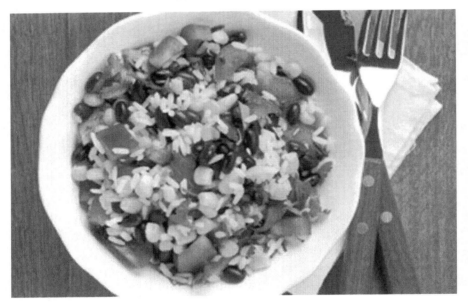

Ingredients:

- 2 cans of black beans
- 1 cup veggie stock
- 1 tablespoon Liquid Aminos
- 1 teaspoon red chili powder
- 2 chopped tomatoes
- 3 chopped green onions
- 1 cup corn
- 2 chopped and seeded green peppers
- 1 bunch cilantro leaves

- 1 avocado
- 3 cups cooked rice
- Salsa to taste

Instructions:

1. Heat the beans with about 2 cups of water, the liquid aminos and chili powder.
2. Serve the rice onto plates. Ladle the beans over the rice according to taste.
3. Add chopped vegetables on top of the rice and beans.
4. Cover with salsa to taste.

Tip: *You can use pinto or kidney beans in place of black beans.*

Nutritional Information: 703 calories per serving, 119g carbs, 10g fat, 39g protein, 30.3g fiber

5| *Mac n' Cheese*

Servings: 6

Prep Time: 20 Minutes
Cook Time: 20 Minutes

Nothing says all-American like a nice warm bowl of Mac n' Cheese. Well, now even us Vegans can enjoy this all-time favorite.

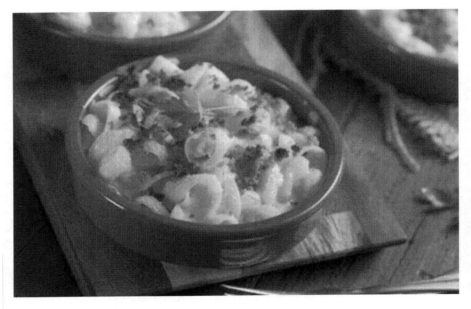

Ingredients:

- 1½ cups raw cashews
- 3 tablespoons lemon juice
- ¾ cup water
- 1½ teaspoon sea salt
- ¼ cup nutritional yeast
- ½ teaspoon chili powder
- ½ clove garlic
- pinch of turmeric

- pinch of cayenne pepper
- ½ teaspoon Dijon mustard
- 8 oz. of elbow or shell pasta of choice

Instructions:

1. Preheat the oven to 350F. Start boiling some water to prepare your pasta. Cook according to package directions.
2. Add the cashews into a blender and blend until they are finely ground. Once the cashews have been processed and are the correct consistency, add the rest of the ingredients and blend until you have a thick smooth consistency.
3. By this point, your pasta should be ready or very close to it. Once it is cooked to your liking, drain and rinse it. Once drained, return it to the pot. Now add the "cheese sauce" and mix well with the pasta. Let it sit on low heat for a couple of minutes to heat the sauce through.
4. Serve while hot and enjoy!

Tip: You can also add veggies to this dish. Some delish sautéed broccoli would make this dish even more amazing.

Nutritional Information: 224 calories per serving, 14.7g carbs, 10g fat, 8.4g protein, 2.9g fiber

6| *Black Bean Veggie Burger*

Servings: 6

Prep Time: 15 Minutes
Cook Time: 35 Minutes

I'm sure you would agree that no collection of vegan recipes would be complete without a vegan burger recipe. Well, here we are giving you a great burger you can cook up in no time.

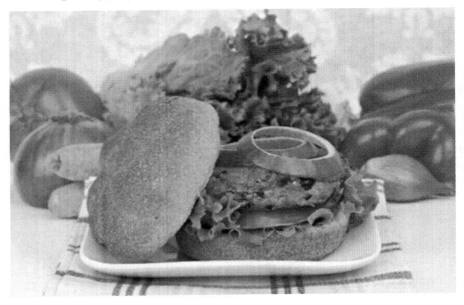

Ingredients:

- 1 red bell pepper
- 5 small red potatoes
- 2 cans black beans, drained and rinsed
- ¾ cup smooth salsa
- 2 teaspoons chili powder
- 1 teaspoon ground cumin
- ¼ cup medium grind coarse cornmeal

Instructions:

1. Preheat oven to 400 degrees.
2. Chop your bell pepper. Make sure to cut it into small pieces so that it will mix easily with the burger batter. Place them onto a sheet pan lined with parchment paper and roast in the oven for about 10 minutes.
3. Peel the potatoes and wrap them in plastic. Cook them in the microwave until they are tender. Alternately, you could roast them, but do NOT boil as boiling will make the burgers mushy. Mash the cooked potatoes and measure out 1 tightly packed cup. Set this aside.
4. Drain and rinse your black beans. Make sure there is no excess water on the beans. Measure out 1 cup of the black beans and place into a large mixing bowl. The rest of the beans should be placed into a food processor. Add the potatoes to the processor as well. Pulse until you have a sticky, thick mashed paste. It should only take a few pulses.
5. Add this mixture to the bowl of extra beans.
6. In a separate small bowl, combine the salsa, chili powder, and cumin and mix well. Pour the salsa mixture over the bowl of beans and potatoes and add the cooked bell pepper.
7. Mix all of the ingredients together until everything is combined well and you have a thick, sticky paste.
8. Lastly, mix the cornmeal into the batter until combined well. Place the batter into the fridge for 30 minutes prior to baking. This will help with forming the patties later on.
9. After chilling, form 6 patties and place them on a sheet pan lined with parchment paper.
10. Bake at 375 degrees for 25 minutes. Remove the pan and using a thin metal spatula carefully flip them. After you have flipped all 6 patties, cook for additional 10 minutes.
11. Remove the patties from the oven and let cool while you prepare your patties and the toppings you will use.

Nutritional Information: 616 calories per serving, 117.6g carbs, 2.7g fat, 34g protein, 25.6g fiber

7| *Tomato Soup*

Servings: varies depending on use

Prep Time: 20 Minutes
Cook Time: 20 Minutes

To round up our delicious lunch section, we are offering you a wonderful and easy-to-prepare soup. This soup is great year round.

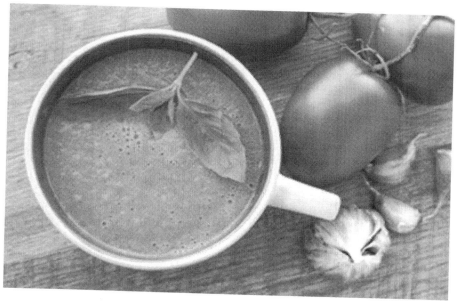

Ingredients:

- 1 onion, diced
- 2 garlic cloves, minced
- 2 tablespoons water
- 4 lbs. ripe tomatoes
- 1 cup vegetable broth
- Cilantro for garnish

Instructions:

1. Prepare a large pot with water and add the diced onion and minced garlic. Cook until they are soft, adding water as necessary.
2. Add the tomatoes (which should be peeled, seeded, and chopped) and broth to the pot. Bring to a boil then reduce heat and simmer for about 15 minutes.
3. Once this is cooked, add to a blender and puree.
4. Serve the soup and garnish with some cilantro or other herb of your choosing.

Nutritional Information: 139 calories per serving, 27.9g carbs, 1.7g fat, 7.5g protein, 8.1g fiber

Dinner

1| *Black Bean Wrap*

Servings: 1

Prep Time: 5 Minutes
Cook Time: 5 Minutes

Let's face it. We don't always want a big elaborate production when it comes to dinner. This wrap will help you serve a dish that is filling and tastes great without all the fuss.

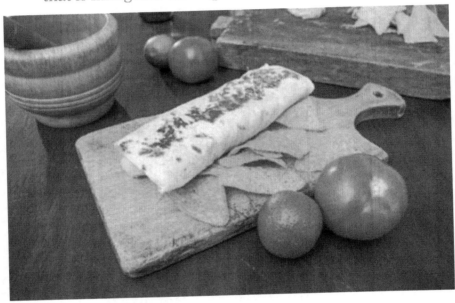

Ingredients:

- 1 large whole grain tortilla
- ⅓ cup salsa
- ¼ cup black beans
- ¼ cup corn
- ¼ avocado, chopped
- 1 large handful of baby greens
- 2 sprigs of cilantro, chopped

Instructions:

1. Warm tortilla using your preferred method.
2. Pour salsa onto the tortilla. It's best to keep to one side in order to make the wrapping part easier.
3. Spread the black beans, corn, and avocado over salsa.
4. Sprinkle the cilantro over the bean mixture and then top with the greens of your choosing.
5. Fold sides of the wrap over the ingredients and then roll from one side to the other. Cut the wrap in half and serve.

Nutritional Information: 269 calories per serving, 34.7g carbs, 10g fat, 11g protein, 10g fiber

2| *Quinoa Teriyaki*

Servings: 4

Prep Time: 5 Minutes
Cook Time: 10 Minutes

This dish is satisfying and the texture of it is amazing. It's chewy and creamy all in one. It'll be a hit at the dinner table.

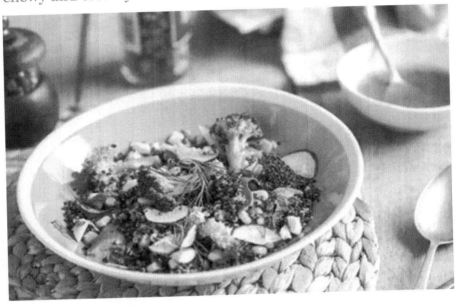

Ingredients:

- 2 large baked sweet potatoes
- 2 cups cooked quinoa
- ¼ cup water
- 4 cups broccoli florets
- 1 small onion
- 1 avocado
- ½ cup teriyaki sauce

Instructions:

1. Add ¼ cup of water to a sauté pan. Add chopped onion, mushrooms and broccoli. Cover and cook on medium high heat for about 10 minutes. Stir occasionally.
2. Warm up the quinoa and sweet potatoes separately in the microwave.
3. When the vegetables are done, add the warmed up quinoa to the sauté pan and stir to mix with vegetables.
4. Serve warmed sweet potatoes into bowls according to servings.
5. Add the quinoa/vegetable mixture right atop of the sweet potatoes and then cover with avocados.
6. Drizzle teriyaki sauce according to taste. Mix lightly and enjoy.

Nutritional Information: 486 calories per serving, 72g carbs, 10g fat, 18g protein, 12g fiber

3| *Shepard's Pie*

Servings: 6

Prep Time: 35 Minutes
Cook Time: 60 Minutes

This Shepard's pie recipe makes me reminisce of my childhood and when I would sit at the table with my family. Create a new memory for your family or friends with the healthy vegan dish.

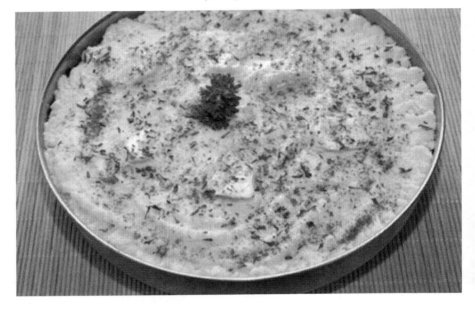

Ingredients:

- 3 cups veggie broth
- 1 chopped onion
- 1 celery stalk
- 1 green pepper
- ½ teaspoon sage leaves
- 1 tablespoon soy sauce
- 1 carrot

- 1 ½ cups cauliflower florets
- 1 cup cabbage
- 1 cup greens beans
- mix of 2 tablespoons cornstarch & 1/3 cup cold water
- pepper to taste
- 3 cups mashed potatoes

Instructions:

1. Preheat oven to 350F.
2. In a large pot, cook ½ cup veggie broth, onion, celery, bell pepper and garlic. Make sure to stir occasionally, for about 4 minutes. Add the sage and soy sauce and stir. Then add the remaining vegetable broth along with the carrots, cauliflower, cabbage and green beans.
3. Bring to a boil and cover, then reduce heat and cook for 20 minutes on low-medium heat.
4. Add the cornstarch mixture and stir until it begins to thicken. Season with pepper to taste.
5. Transfer to a casserole dish and cover vegetable mixture with mashed potatoes. Bake for 30 minutes or until potatoes are slightly browned.

Nutritional Information: 127 calories per serving, 25.5g carbs, 1.6g fat, 4g protein, 2g fiber

4| *Vegetable Pasta*

Servings: 4-6

Prep Time: 15 Minutes
Cook Time: 15 Minutes

This one-pot pasta recipe will be the recipe that will keep on giving. Why? Substitute different vegetables and pasta sauce every time you make it and will be like a whole new dish each time.

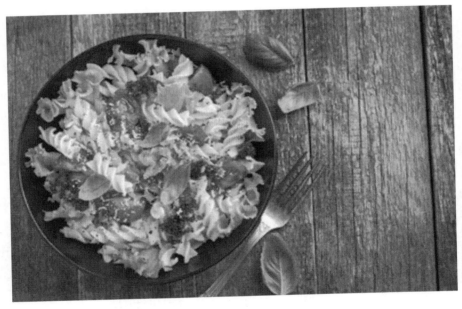

Ingredients:

- 1 lb. pasta (preferably wholegrain)
- 2 cups broccoli florets
- bunch of spinach
- cherry tomatoes
- 1 jar of your favorite pasta sauce

Instructions:

1. Cook pasta in a large pot according to package directions.
2. In a separate pot, cook vegetables according to preferred softness.
3. Drain the pasta and vegetables then add everything into one pot and mix with pasta sauce.

Nutritional Information: 245 calories per serving, 46.2g carbs, 2g fat, 11g protein, 2g fiber

5| *Lasagna Rolls*

Servings: 5

Prep Time: 10 Minutes
Cook Time: 25 Minutes

Lasagna is one of my favorite dinner dishes. It's great for dinner parties or for a few guests. Cook up a batch and serve this at your next get-together or for a simple family meal.

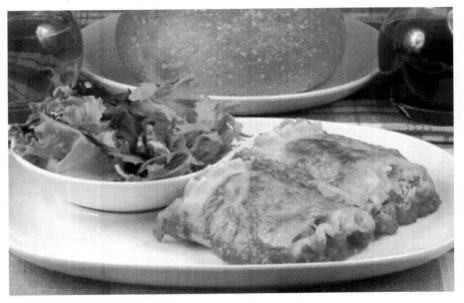

Ingredients:

- lasagna noodles
- 2 ripe avocados
- 2 tablespoons vegan Parmesan
- ¼ teaspoon garlic powder
- 2 teaspoon basil
- 1/3 cup chopped baby spinach leaves
- 1 tablespoon parsley
- 6 grape tomatoes

- pepper to taste
- ½ cup sauce

Instructions:

1. Preheat oven to 350F.
2. Cook about 5 lasagna noodles according to package directions.
3. Combine to avocado, Parmesan, garlic powder, basil, spinach, parsley, tomatoes and pepper. Mix all these ingredients until they are well combined.
4. In a baking dish, cover the bottom with marinara sauce.
5. Take one lasagna noodle and place it on a clean flat surface. Spread some of the mixture across the entire length of the noodle. Roll up the noodle and place upright into the baking dish. Repeat this for all the noodles.
6. Cover the dish with aluminum foil and bake for 20 minutes.

Nutritional Information: 281 calories per serving, 23g carbs, 17g fat, 5g protein, 9g fiber

6| *Tortilla Casserole*

Servings: 6

Prep Time: 15 Minutes
Cook Time: 15 Minutes

This casserole is a one-dish wonder. You can have dinner ready on the table in 30 minutes! Great for those long days.

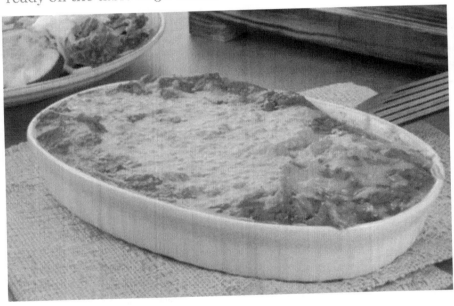

Ingredients:

- 1 can black beans, drained and rinsed
- 1 can diced tomatoes
- 1 can chopped mild green chilies
- 2 cups corn kernels
- 1 bunch scallions, chopped
- 1 teaspoon chili powder
- 1 teaspoon ground cumin
- ½ teaspoon dried oregano
- 12 corn tortillas

- 2 cups vegan cheese
- Salsa

Instructions:

1. Preheat oven to 400° F.
2. Combine beans, tomatoes, chilies, corn, scallions, chili powder, cumin, and oregano in a bowl.
3. Line the bottom of a casserole dish with 6 tortillas, allowing them to overlap in the middle. Scoop on half of the bean mixture and sprinkle on half of the cheese. Add another layer of tortillas as you did before and add the rest of the bean mixture and the rest of the cheese.
4. Bake in the oven for 12-15 minutes.
5. Cut into squares and serve with your favorite salsa.

Nutritional Information: 396 calories per serving, 77g carbs, 2.9g fat, 19g protein, 15.6g fiber

7| *Chickpea Chili*

Servings: 6

Prep Time: 35 Minutes
Cook Time: 45 Minutes

This chili is a great comfort dish everyone will love. It will be worth the wait, guaranteed.

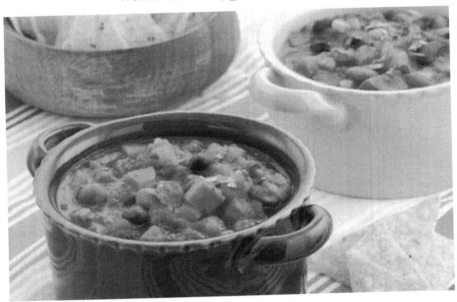

Ingredients:

- 1 diced onion
- 2 garlic cloves, minced
- 1 diced jalapeño
- 2 cans chickpeas
- 1 can of creamy white bean of choice
- 1 can diced green chiles (=chilies)
- 1½ teaspoon cumin
- 1 teaspoon dried thyme
- ¼ teaspoon pepper

- 1 teaspoon oregano
- 1 teaspoon smoked paprika
- 1 teaspoon chili powder
- 3 cups vegetable stock
- 1 cup corn

Instructions:

1. In a pot sauté the onion, garlic and jalapeño over medium heat for 5 minutes.
2. Add the beans, diced green chiles and all the spices. Mix everything well. Stir in the broth and simmer for 20-30 minutes.
3. Add the corn and let simmer for about 2-3 minutes longer.
4. Serve hot with your favorite toppings.

Nutritional Information: 35 calories per serving, 8g carbs, 0.5g fat, 1.2g protein, 1.5g fiber

Dessert (Healthier Options)

Recipes Included in this Chapter:

1| Peach Cobbler

2| Raw Apple Crumble

3| Dark Chocolate Brownies

4| Piña Colada Smoothie

5| Chocolate Mousse

6| Banana Cream Pie

7| Apple Strudel

1| *Peach Cobbler*

Servings: 1

Prep Time: 5 Minutes
Cook Time: 2 Minutes

This peach cobbler is so easy it will take you all of seven minutes to make. Break this out after a great dinner and everyone will think you slaved all day making this treat.

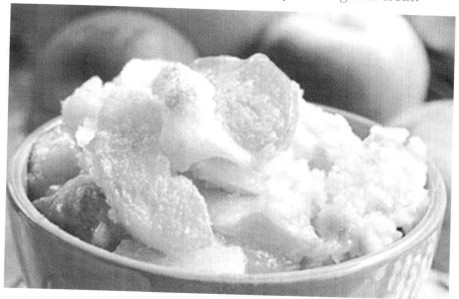

Ingredients:

- 1 peach, sliced
- 1 tablespoon white whole-wheat flour
- 2 tablespoons instant oats
- 1 tablespoon brown sugar
- A pinch ground cinnamon
- A pinch ground nutmeg
- 1 tablespoon nondairy milk
- 1 tablespoon vanilla vegan yogurt

Instructions:

1. Place peaches in a mug and set aside
2. In a small bowl, whisk flour, instant oats, brown sugar, a pinch of ground cinnamon and a pinch of ground nutmeg.
3. Stir in nondairy milk.
4. Pour the oat mixture on top of the peaches and microwave 1–2 minutes, until the oat topping looks a little like oatmeal.
5. Serve hot with your favorite toppings.

Nutritional Information: 126 calories per serving, 28.5g carbs, 0.9g fat, 2.7g protein, 2.7g fiber

2| *Raw Apple Crumble*

Servings: 4

Prep Time: 15 Minutes
Cook Time: 0 Minutes

This is a great desert to make because it requires no baking. The flavors come from whole foods and not bad-for-you additives.

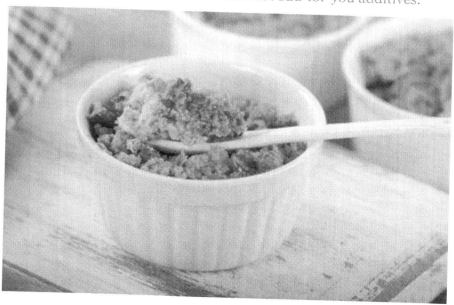

Ingredients:

- 1 cup walnuts
- 4 pitted dates
- 5 apples, largely diced
- 3 tablespoon lemon juice
- 6 pitted Medjool dates
- ¼ teaspoon cinnamon
- ¼ teaspoon nutmeg

Instructions:

1. Starting with the topping, blend the walnuts and 4 dates in a blender or food processor. Transfer this mix into a small bowl.
2. Moving on to the filling, toss 3 apples with 1 tablespoon of lemon juice and set aside.
3. Place the remaining 2 chopped apples into a blender or food processor and blend along with 2 tablespoons of lemon juice, 6 pitted dates, cinnamon and nutmeg.
4. Once blended, pour it onto the apples you set aside and toss.
5. Serve the filling in small dessert dishes and cover with the date-nut topping.

Tip: *Some good suggestions as to what apples to use are Gala or Fiji.*

Nutritional Information: 339 calories per serving, 41g carbs, 10g fat, 8g protein, 8g fiber

3| *Dark Chocolate Brownies*

Servings: 20

Prep Time: 15 Minutes
Cook Time: 20 Minutes

Honestly, is there anything better than a nice moist, chocolatey brownie? Didn't think so. These brownies are chewy, rich and fudgey and best of all-vegan!

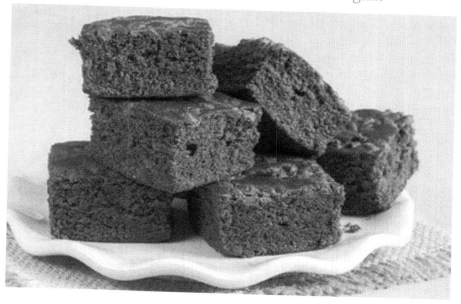

Ingredients:

- ¼ cup pureed avocado
- 1 cup white whole-wheat flour
- ½ cup unsweetened cocoa powder
- ¾ cup cane sugar
- 1 teaspoon baking soda
- ½ teaspoon salt
- ¾ cup water

- 1 ½ cups vegan semisweet chocolate chips

Instructions:

1. Preheat oven to 350F.
2. In a large mixing bowl, mix together the pureed avocado, flour, cocoa powder, sugar, baking soda, salt and water. Stir all of the ingredients until smooth. Fold in 1 cup of the chocolate chips.
3. Pour into a nonstick baking pan creating an even layer. Sprinkle with an additional ½ cup of chocolate chips on top. Bake for 15-20 minutes.
4. Let cool and serve.

Nutritional Information: 30 calories per serving, 5.8g carbs, 0.8g fat, 1.3g protein, 1.5g fiber

4| *Piña Colada Smoothie*

Servings: 1

Prep Time: 5 Minutes
Cook Time: 5 Minutes

This smoothie will have you dreaming of beaches and sunshine. It's smooth and tasty, with none of the bad stuff.

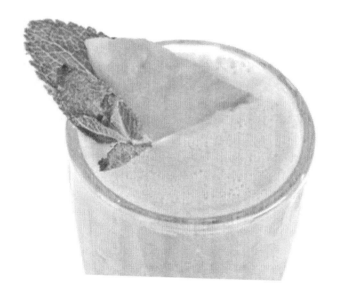

Ingredients:

- 1 Frozen Banana
- 1 Cup Pineapple
- 1¼ Cup Rice Milk
- 1 teaspoon Coconut Extract
- ¼ teaspoon Vanilla Extract

Instructions:

1. Add all the ingredients into a blender and blend!

Tip: When a recipe calls for coconut milk you can use coconut extract added to rice or almond milk.

Nutritional Information: 190 calories per serving, 48.8g carbs, 0.6g fat, 2.2g protein, 5.4g fiber

5| *Chocolate Mousse*

Servings: 2

Prep Time: 5 Minutes
Cook Time: 5 Minutes

This mousse is great for when you are having a chocolate craving. This healthier mousse recipe is rich, creamy and satisfying.

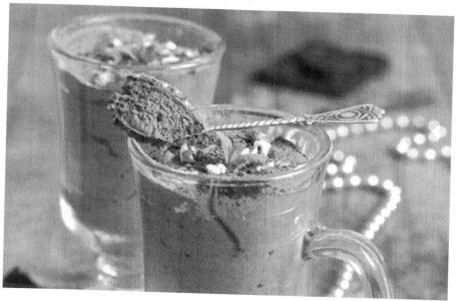

Ingredients:

- 1 ½ cups rice milk
- 6 tablespoons unsweetened cocoa
- ¼ teaspoon peppermint extract
- vegan chocolate chips

Instructions:

1. Whisk together all three ingredients until you begin to

see air bubbles appear.

2. Pour into small dessert bowls or ramekins and place into fridge to set, preferably overnight.

3. Once mousse has set, sprinkle on some chocolate chips and serve.

Nutritional Information: 129 calories per serving, 27.5g carbs, 3.7g fat, 3.5g protein, 5.4g fiber

6| *Banana Cream Pie*

Servings: 6

Prep Time: 1 hour 45 Minutes

These banana cream pies may be mini, but they pack a delicious punch. This recipe combines the goodness of bananas, peanut butter and chocolate chips into wonderful small hand held package.

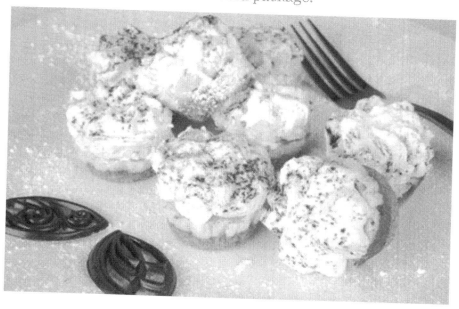

Ingredients:

- ½ cup large pitted medjool dates
- ½ cup sunflower butter
- ¼ cup ground flax seed
- ½ cup dry rolled oats
- 2 tablespoons water
- 1 cup cashews
- 1 large ripe banana
- ¼ tablespoon vanilla

- ¼ teaspoon fine sea salt
- 2 tablespoons lemon juice
- 1 tablespoon water

Instructions:

1. To begin working on the crust, add dates into a bowl and cover with boiling water. Let soak for 15 minutes then drain.
2. Add the dates, peanut butter, flax seed, rolled oats and 2 tablespoons of water to a food processor or a blender.
3. Pulse the ingredients until they start to clump together.
4. Use a spatula to scrape the mixture into a bowl. Roll the mixture into 6 dough balls.
5. Line a muffin tin with six small sheets of plastic wrap, then place a dough ball in each lined cup.
6. Press down the center of the dough and work it out towards the edges of the cup until it covers the cup in a thin layer.
7. Place the crusts in the refrigerator and move on to work on the filling.
8. Place cashews into a bowl and cover with boiling water. Allow to soak for 30 minutes then drain.
9. Add cashews, banana, vanilla, lemon, salt and water to a cleaned food processer.
10. Blend on high until mixture is creamy.
11. Remove the crust from the refrigerator. Spoon the filling into each crust and refrigerate for at least one hour before serving.
12. Once the pies have set remove them from the tin by pulling up on the plastic wrap. Carefully remove the plastic wrap and serve.

Nutritional Information: 205 calories per serving, 18.8g carbs, 12g fat, 5.6g protein, 3.2g fiber

7| *Apple Strudel*

Servings: 1

Prep Time: 5 Minutes
Cook Time: 15 Minutes

This recipe for a traditional Austrian dessert can be made using only 3 ingredients. It's perfect for a quick dessert or to show off some baking skills for some guests.

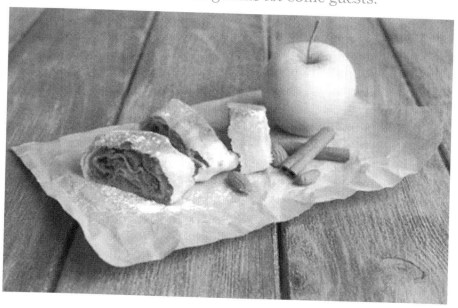

Ingredients:

- 1 package vegan puff pastry dough
- 2 apples
- ¾ teaspoon cinnamon

Instructions:

1. Pre-heat oven to 350°F.
2. Remove the pastry dough from the refrigerator and allow to thaw.

3. Peel the apples and get rid of the seeds.
4. Slice the apples into very thin slices.
5. Add the cinnamon to the apple slices and mix well.
6. Place the apples onto the pastry dough (which should now be on a baking pan) and fold it in then close the edges.
7. Place the apple strudel into the oven and bake for about 15 minutes.
8. Once the strudel is finished baking, serve.

Nutritional Information: 194 calories per serving, 51g carbs, 0.7g fat, 1g protein, 9.7g fiber

Conclusion

Hopefully these vegan recipes will help you to create a meal plan that will keep you on track. Remember that all of the recipes can be altered to suit your tastes, just make sure to keep within the "guidelines". Clean eating can be fun and delicious, so give these recipes a try.

So what are you waiting for, start cooking!

Your Exclusive Gift

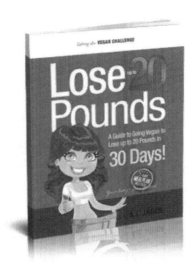

Fit in Your Jeans!

As a „Thank you" for downloading this book I would like to give you my eBook: *Lose up to 20 Pounds in 30 Days!* for FREE. This is a no strings attached offer.

Based on Scientific Research

Say goodbye to those unhealthy and untested crash diets and fad diets and say hello to the scientifically proven, healthy, and effective vegan diet. Get this book today and get ready to make a change in your life that will actually make a difference!

You'll not only get the facts about going vegan but real, practical tips for making the change in your own life. If you're worried about breaking the budget, this book offers you a fully nutritious, 100% vegan diet plan for just $35 per week. You may have stumbled upon the vegan diet in hopes of losing weight. On that count, you will not be disappointed. When done right, the vegan diet can help you lose all those unwanted pounds quickly and safely. And this book will help you do it right.

Typical results of a low-fat starch-based vegan diet:

• A healthy weight loss
• A healthier body
• More energy
• Healthy skin
• Alleviation of allergy symptoms
• Significant reduction of body odor
• Healthier hair and stronger nails
• Relief from migraines
• Revert Diabetes Type 2
• Longer life

Visit www.ybyf.gr8.com to Get Your FREE eBook Now!

NEW – Available Now

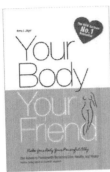

The NEW German No. 1 Bestseller:
Your Body, Your Friend

The Answer to Permanently Becoming Slim, Healthy, and Happy
Based on Scientific Research

Fat Storer Goodbye!
Fat Burner Hello.

In the course of her research, bestselling author and long-time nutritionist Anna I. Jäger discovered a fairly simple, logical solution: We need to stop fighting against the biologically natural processes of the organism that we call our bodies. We need to, instead, join forces with them! A healthy, well nourished body will run more efficiently and lose its extra pounds automatically.

No, these are not false promises; this is biology.

Your Body Needs Energy to Heal
Your Body Needs Energy to Feel Happy
Your Body Needs Energy to Burn Fat (!)

As you read through these chapters, you'll learn:

- How to train your body to become a fat burner, not a fat storer
- Why cutting calories is dangerous for your mind and body
- Why low carb diets will make you gain more fat longterm
- How to overcome an eating disorder
- How to lower your set-point (the weight your body tries to maintain)

Make Your Body Your Powerful Ally

Get this book so you can learn how you can transform your body and life starting today by becoming best friends with your body and nourishing yourself into a new, slim, healthy, and happy you!

ISBN-13: 978-1508525448
ISBN-10: 1508525447

86

Recommendations

Recommended books on nutrition:

T. Colin Campbell, Thomas M. Campbell
The China Study
The Most Comprehensive Study of Nutrition Ever Conducted And the Startling Implications for Diet, Weight Loss, And Long-term Health

Dr. John A. McDougall, MD
The Starch Solution
Eat the foods you love, regain your health, and lose the weight for good

Dr. Neal Bernard, MD
Power Foods for the Brain
An Effective 3-Step Plan to Protect Your Mind and Strengthen Your Memory
21-Day Weight Loss Kickstart
Boost Metabolism, Lower Cholesterol, and Dramatically Improve Your Health
Dr. Neal Barnard's Program for Reversing Diabetes
The Scientifically Proven System for Reversing Diabetes without Drugs

Dr. Caldwell B. Esselstyn Jr.
Prevent and Reverse Heart Disease
The Revolutionary, Scientifically Proven, Nutrition-Based Cure

Copyright & Legal Information

"Vegan Cookbook for Beginners
Transform Your Life!
Fat-Free Quick & Easy Vegan Recipes
Delicious Recipes Purely Starch-Plant Based for a Dairy-Free, Low-Cholesterol, Low-Fat Diet"
by Jäger, Anna I.
Series: Low-Fat Vegan Cooking Recipe Book (3)
Published by:
Anna I. Jäger
Red. Guer, Engelthaler Str., 60435 Frankfurt am Main, Germany
First Edition February 2016 (Version 1.1)

Inquiries: ivijaeger@gmail.com

Updated February 4th, 2016

Image rights:
Fotolia.com:
65785780 © Africa Studio, 88011580 © pristineimages, 73540587 © lilechka75, 67021581 © Ruslan Olinchuk, 78950781 © dreamon512, 99512970 © bit24, 54651001 © Stephanie Frey, 65394859 © fotogal, 41433241 © MSPhotographic, 20561436 © rafer76, 81674622 © anna_shepulova, 51175960 © Bill, 87125842 © vanillaechoes, 64810102 © Fotos 593, 70125683 © gekaskr, 87346222 © RoJo Images, 66809294 © Brent Hofacker, 79617680 © mariashumova, 16358837 © JJAVA, 56779576 © denio109, 99193089 © natalieina17, 79260217 © istetiana, 88290784 © Yulia Furman, 92627116 © Jenifoto, 87914396 © azurita, 84131594 © bit24, 83191710 © olepeshkina, 81141236 © Boyarkina Marina, 55267435 © cristi lucaci, 79967488 © minadezhda, 91787024 © 5second, 77605248 © dbvirago, 86118110 © bit24, 69142051 © Brent Hofacker, 87962221 © epitavi

Made in the USA
San Bernardino, CA
28 January 2017